Part one : The art of healthy eating

Appolinaire LIMA

CONTENTS

INTRODUCTION

For a few reasons, certainly considered one among the toughest matters for a human to do is to devour proper. Whether this is due to the fact we've got constrained to get right of entry to sources in all regions or if it's miles due to the fact we definitely have an excessive amount of get right of entry to bad meals, there are numerous motives that ingesting healthful food is a challenge.

Sure, we are able to devour pretty much whatever, and it's going to preserve us. We will control transport from one second to the next and have the ability to name ourselves healthy. Is it unhealthy to eat sugary drinks? Just due to the fact we're alive does now no longer suggest that we're healthy. And the older we get, the greater our awful conduct starts to capture up with us.

Shape healthy eating habits early in life, or at least, as early as possible save you from future problems. All folks want to take greater obligation or responsibility ace into our bodies, due to the fact if we fact that, it may turn out to be extraordinarily dangerous.
Of course, whilst we recognize we're capable of returning to our mistakes, hindsight is 20/20. We , and that there have been matters that we ought to have carried out and likely need to have carried out that we definitely didn't do due to the fact we have been both subconscious of the unwell results, or definitely lazy. Just having the easy information does now no longer always cause them to want to do something fitness aware.

For the maximum part, it takes us genuinely being uncovered to the struggles that could arise due to awful fitness selections earlier than we're greater aware of the manner we deal with our bodies and our fitness in general. When we aren't capable of see the truth of the outcomes to our actions, it may cause them to feel recognize a long way away and tough to narrate to. We may also even blow them off entirely. This may be a completely debilitating vicinity to discover yourself in. Especially whilst you are already dealing from the facet results of bad ingesting and a loss of a healthful eating regimen.

It is always difficult to accept and endure change. Also, switching to a vegetarian diet is not as easy as you might think, so it is very important to do a thorough analysis before adapting to a new lifestyle. Sometimes transitioning to a meatless diet can be difficult, so it's best to know the ins and outs beforehand, because becoming a vegetarian means a lot more than just giving up meat. There are different types of vegetarians, some prefer to eat fish and others don't. On the other hand, there are people who don't even consume dairy products, including cheese and eggs, and subsist on fruits and vegetables. Switching to a vegetarian diet is always an individual preference. Supplements that the body needs should also be considered before avoiding cottage cheese and other nutritious foods that provide important nutrients. It is best to start slowly with and gradually become a total vegetarian.

Although it may be hard to believe, the entire body system will experience definite changes as the body is not getting something it has become very accustomed to. It is always better to gradually reduce the amount. Rather than suddenly eliminating meat from your routine diet, replace it with intake of fish or chicken and then begin to gradually reduce consumption by gradually becoming a full vegetarian. The most important part of becoming a vegetarian is knowing the contents of foods that would be eaten instead of meat. In general, those who do not approve of a vegetarian lifestyle assume that if meat were not added to the diet, their bodies would be deprived of essential vitamins and minerals.

However, there are many who have successfully transitioned to a meatless diet. These people were able to provide their bodies with the necessary nutrients and thus fill in the backlog of the meatless diet. Extensive research has shown that green vegetables like broccoli, kale, and spinach contain tremendous amounts of calcium, and consuming these green vegetables would provide the nutrients you need to stay healthy. Walnuts are also known to be a rich source of protein. You get enough to live a healthy life with a balanced diet.

Switching to a vegetarian diet is one of the most important things you can do to keep your body feeling healthy. And for people who have already converted to a vegan lifestyle, they must have found that they feel great and have excess energy and have also been able to lose weight without starving. So think about it and move towards a fulfilling lifestyle.

Everybody merits a threat to turn out to be the finest model of themselves viable, however if we aren't even acknowledging the truth that bad ingesting can take us properly off course, even Very the gift second, then we're in the end waving inside to the great destiny.

But all of this will change. By analyzing this book, you will apprehend the significance of ingesting health and the way meals influence our bodies and functions.

Without understanding exactly why our bodies respond the way we do to food, it can sometimes be difficult to stay on track. Start a healthy eating journey. Don't waste any more time. We should start eating healthy today!

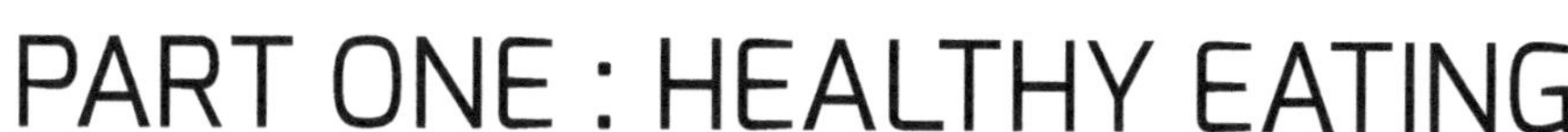

PART ONE : HEALTHY EATING

CHAPTER 1: WHY EAT HEALTHY?

Healthy eating is important for many reasons. Most of us are already aware of the growing obesity epidemic in North America. This is especially true in the United States in general. The term for the way many Americans eat is called the SAD diet.

SAD stands for Standard American Diet and refers to a diet low in vegetables, high in fat and sugar and deficient in nutrients. Processed foods are definitely a part of the SAD diet. These are foods that are readily available and quick to consume and prepare, but have long-lasting negative health effects. If you don't want to become obese, it's generally considered a good idea to avoid eating such processed foods and focus on eating whole grains, fruits and vegetables, and meats that aren't treated with hormones and other chemicals that can eventually end up in your body and cause problems. Unfortunately, in North America, we have many opportunities to slack off when it comes to meal preparation.

We have so many things at our disposal, and we have to spend far less money to buy bad food than to buy good food. It seems odd that buying organic foods costs more money than buying foods that ultimately lead to long-term health problems, but that's the rule of supply and demand. Not only that, processed foods are mass-produced and make a huge profit because of their convenience. For this reason, the obesity epidemic in North America is not particularly surprising in many respects. Nutrition isn't number one on the list of companies trying to capitalize on people's laziness in the kitchen.

However, there are many reasons why a healthy diet is important and good reasons to avoid processed foods and the standard American diet. For example, if you don't want to become obese, you should definitely read the rest of this book. To find ways to improve your diet and start a healthier lifestyle. Another reason to eat healthy is that you can make yourself susceptible to disease by eating unhealthy foods and following a standard American diet that is loaded with fat and sugar. Diabetes is something that can develop from a poor diet and can often be treated with a healthy diet. Ultimately, Type II diabetes is something that can be maintained and controlled by proper eating habits and triggered by poor eating habits.

If you want to avoid these kinds of pitfalls and complications, you should do your best to be mindful of your food choices.

Other diseases can also result from a poor diet. Hypertension is common, as are other chronic diseases. You may find that you suffer from poor bone health, high blood pressure, or even heart problems. All of this can put a lot of strain on your body and cause great stress, which can ultimately be very dangerous.

If you want to show your family that you care, you must start making decisions now that will help you stay in their lives as long as possible. Illness is not something that only affects you. Something that affects the people around you. When they see you suffering because of the bad choices you made, that's pretty selfish in a way. They suffer too.

Do your best now to make the best decisions, not just for yourself, but for your family in the long run. This book will show you how.

CHAPTER 2: UNDERSTANDING YOUR FOOD RELATIONSHIP

Everyone, over time, develops certain behaviors. We form habits in many aspects of our life. We form hygiene habits, food habits, work habits, and a variety of other habits. However, people frequently do not notice our tendencies until it is too late.

Begin to wreak havoc on us. Even when we see that our behaviors are negatively impacting us, altering them can be challenging. Because that's the way I like it. A habit is something we do nearly instinctively. We are conditioned to follow these routines, and breaking the loop requires a lot of effort.

Once you begin to understand that your relationship with food has **a lot** to do with the habits you have **formed** and **the** habits you can continue to **form** and cultivate, it becomes **much** easier to change **the way** you **think. When you recognize** the impact and importance of your **future,** and make positive **decisions** about **those** things, **you** can **better prepare for** healthy eating and **be** less inclined to make **decisions** that negatively impact you and your **future.**

To be honest, many of us appear to be pessimistic about the future. We don't see enough reasons to modify our habits because if we don't feel we have something positive to look forward to, it makes no difference whether we make good choices or not. We don't see how we can shape our future in our best interests. Most likely

because we do not think we have any control over our life.
Don't be frightened if you recognize this sensation. It is quite prevalent in human experience. We are normally discouraged from taking charge and exercising our power from a young age, and we may have given up believing we have any influence over our life because we are frequently told what to do by others.
That makes sense for youngsters. Children are not always aware of what is best for them. However, it may foster a powerless perspective, making it difficult to appreciate how the repercussions of our choices can genuinely begin to define who we are and how we show ourselves to the world.
This is why it is critical to take genuine measures to better understand yourself and your food habits. When did you start doing it? How did you develop that habit? Why? What advantages does this behavior provide you? What are the negative consequences of this practice for you?

Ask yourself as many of these questions as you can so that you may begin to genuinely comprehend how the food you consume is creating your future. Are you seeing a future that is healthy and energized, or one that is dark and perhaps full of bad health consequences?
Next, assess your sense of self-control. Are you capable of exercising self-control over your choices? Is this an area in which you struggle? Discipline may be tough for everyone, and if you are having difficulty keeping disciplined, you should look into numerous methods that you can urge yourself to be a more disciplined person, both physically and psychologically.

Only then will you actually have what it takes to go on a healthy eating path. Because, whether we like it or not, poor health decisions are all around us. They are simple and addictive.
If we allow ourselves to be misled by these poor choices and do nothing to improve our behaviors, it makes little difference whether we eat healthily occasionally or not. The harmful consequences will continue to grip your body and surprise you

when you least expect it.

In some ways, unhealthy eating is a self-destructive practice in which many of us engage. Self-destructive eating behaviors are harmful, whether they are caused by low self-esteem or simply because we are unhappy with our circumstances and have lost trust in the future. Before eating healthy to stay, you must first look to yourself and sincerely respect your life and future.

There are several methods to do this, and if feasible, you should seek the assistance of a mental health expert. They can sometimes help us recognize biases and unfavorable tendencies in our life that we are unaware of. Once things are acknowledged and accepted, it may be much simpler to overcome them and take the necessary measures to make great choices.
Whether you seek the assistance of a competent expert or not, there are several things you can do to alter your thinking. As long as you believe you are deserving of a healthy body and a bright future, you will be willing to take the required efforts to get there.

It will be much more difficult if you do not feel good about yourself. Overall, recognizing yourself, your habits, mental hurdles, and discipline will assist you on your journey. Every day, we can take steps toward being our best selves, and healthy eating is a terrific place to start. And it's a move we can take right now!

CHAPITRE 3: THE RISKS OF DIET TRENDS

Diet trends abound in our culture today, and virtually all of them are fraught with risk. Unfortunately, most people who are anxious for money do not consider the long-term health implications of their products. What they genuinely care about is generating money and developing something that will allow them to profit off the urgent need that many people have to lose weight quickly and easily.

If diet trends pique your attention, you'll have to accept one thing. Unfortunately, there is no good technique to lose weight quickly and simply without doing any work, eating properly, or exercising. Losing weight is a fantastic objective if you are fat or lack fitness and want greater mobility.
We are all required to start making better lifestyle choices at some point, and that is something we can achieve with food and good body activity rather than by trusting corporations who want to abuse us in order to earn money.

Some food fads are extremely harmful and can have serious long-term and short-term health implications. Many of them rely on technologies that deprive us and our bodies of crucial nutrients. Even dehydrating us at times.

These diet trends are just revolting. They take advantage of those who want to be healthy but don't know where to start. They prey on people, generally women, who are breaking under the strains of artificial beauty standards, and on women who are persuaded that in order to be valuable, they must appear in a specific way. That is just false. You have worth whether you weigh 100 pounds or 700 pounds. Healthy eating, on the other hand, is one of the few genuine methods to jumpstart your metabolism and give your body the nutrition it requires to perform at its best.

If you deprive your body of the vitamins and minerals it requires to survive and trust a diet fad to teach you how to lose weight and have worth when all they actually want is your money, you will finish up more behind than you started. The terrible reality is that many diet trends induce the body to go into famine mode.

This can disrupt your metabolism and cause you to acquire weight more quickly in the future. Allow yourself to be taken advantage of by commercials promising quick and effortless weight loss. All of this will come at a cost. Not only that, but some health trends, such as the HCG diet, can seriously harm your body and hormones.

The irony of diet trends is that they frequently make it more difficult to lose weight in the future, since you are using unhealthy and challenging methods of weight maintenance. If you want to be slim, don't put your faith in a medication advertised on TV. Begin by eliminating harmful sugary and processed meals and replacing them with nutritious whole-grain wheat and organic fruits and veggies that will not introduce chemicals into your body, making it even more difficult to lose weight and eventually messing up your body chemistry.

It may appear appealing to be able to reduce weight rapidly without having to forsake the bad eating habits you have acquired over time, but this is not healthy. If you do not use caution when attempting to reduce weight, you will injure yourself and prime your body for future health concerns. Make certain that you are doing all in your ability to make decisions that you would like others to make for themselves.

Do your homework before succumbing to the snake oil seller on TV. Investigate these matters because you are worth doing things correctly, and you deserve a bright future that is not complicated by the side effects of a sales pitch that just wants your money and not your health.

CHAPTER 4 : THE FOOD PYRAMID

The food pyramid is certainly familiar to most of us. The food pyramid was frequently used as a guideline for us as children to give us an idea of how much food and what type of food we should consume every day in order to maintain a healthy lifestyle.

Of course, there is always data to suggest that the food pyramid is flexible, but observing the food pyramid will give you a basic notion of what is appropriate in a balanced and nutritious diet.
While this might be contentious at times, having basic nourishment is still beneficial. Perhaps one that you designed yourself. Many individuals would argue that eating as many grains as the food pyramid suggests is no longer the healthiest thing to do.

In fact, with recent outbreaks of celiac disease, many individuals are promoting a no-grain lifestyle as the healthiest option.
Rather than depending on the food pyramid as a basic guideline for what is good to eat, try to examine your own particular eating experiences and proceed from there. Some people are healthier when they eat a lot of grains, whereas others are not. Use your best judgment here to the best of your ability so that you can take the proper actions for your health.

The conventional food pyramid suggests the following :
•If you are not allergic or lactose intolerant, you can have two or three portions of their eggs every day.
• It is advised that you have two or three portions of meat and

beans every day, as well as nuts, fish, and chicken.
Surprisingly, sugar, fat, and oil are at the very top of the list. Because none of these things should be in excess. Rather, utilize them just as needed to maintain the best possible lifestyle.

Once again, this is only a reference to the traditional food pyramid. You may need to adapt this chart for yourself based on your own needs and dietary functions. However, if you do not have any special criteria, this is the food pyramid norm that may be used to your maximum advantage in developing a healthy lifestyle.

CHAPTER 5: HOW CAN FOOD BE YOUR MEDICINE?

Similarly to how not eating healthily may make you sick, eating nutritious meals can frequently treat illness and bring relief when you are suffering.

It can also be used as a prophylactic step against disease. In truth, Ayurveda is a medical system that has been practiced for thousands of years in India.

This traditional treatment method is used to treat any condition by just altering your diet. Food is actually the medication that has kept the Indian people alive for millennia. And it may still be relevant today.

Many cures, in reality, are just nutritious meals with anti-inflammatory characteristics and the capacity to nourish your body from the inside. Healthy eating habits have been shown to have an influence on anything from illness to cancer.

And that has never been more evident than with this ancient healing technique.

Of course, most current technology will look down on these ways since they haven't been properly explored, but much of it has been tried and true for thousands of years and will continue to have an influence on the body.

Whether you believe in the ancient healing art or not, the reality remains that diet can ultimately decide your susceptibility to sickness. If you eat correctly, your body will be stronger and better equipped to fight off disease and infection than if you starved on a conventional American diet.

It can be nearly impossible to fight off the bad consequences of disease without the right vitamins and minerals in your body.

It can even cause disease at times. Certain sorts of bad unprocessed foods might really cause diseases and make you more susceptible to certain types of cancer if you consume them.

Although cancer is still being investigated and the scientific world does not completely understand it well enough to cure it, there are many examples of people who were able to live long and healthy lives merely by altering the way they needed to. Healthy nutrition can help reduce the symptoms of many tough and incurable conditions, such as multiple sclerosis.

They will continue to do so as long as you ensure that everything you put into your body is nutritious and provides your organs and cells with all of the fuel and resources they require to keep your body robust. They will perform to the best of their abilities.

However, if you are intentionally destroying your body, it will not be able to fight back as well as it would if it was receiving appropriate nutrients. That is why it is critical that you pay attention to how you fuel your body. If you do not make active and mindful eating choices, you may be setting yourself up for failure in ways that you will live to regret.

CHAPTER 6: VEGETABLE HEALTH BENEFITS

Vegetables are one of the most underappreciated foods in the world, particularly in the conventional American diet. Most individuals underestimate the importance of providing the body with vitamins and minerals that veggies and vegetables alone can give. People will sometimes look into veggies to improve their looks, but when it comes to enhancing their health, they get indifferent.

However, given that you are here and reading this book, it is reasonable to presume that you are ready and able to explore why eating veggies is vital. Here are some of the top reasons to include veggies in your diet on a regular basis.

First and foremost, the body needs fiber to eliminate waste. Without a method to collect and discharge waste, it accumulates in the body, contributing to weight gain and other possible issues. Fiber is also essential for a variety of additional reasons. It can help you keep your blood cholesterol from increasing and potentially prevent or reduce your risks of developing heart disease.

Folic acid is also found in vegetables, and when you consume it, it stimulates the development of red blood cells in your body. This can be quite helpful in preventing anemia and can be especially advantageous to women, who have a predisposition to require this ingredient during pregnancy and menstruation.

Vegetables are also naturally high in numerous vitamins, such as A and C, which aid in infection resistance and overall health. It can help you speed up the healing process and absorb iron, which is another strategy to help battle and avoid anemia. Vitamins are abundant in potassium, which is beneficial since it keeps the body from developing high blood pressure.

Vegetables have been shown to lower the risk of strokes and other cardiovascular problems. They can prevent the formation of kidney stones as well as the degradation of bone materials. Consuming enough of veggies will help you control type II diabetes and weight.

Not only that, but it may assist you in remaining strong in the battle against cancer and in cancer prevention. One of the most appealing aspects of eating veggies is that they are low in fat and low in calories.
This means you may eat as many veggies as you want without worrying about gaining too much weight. Snacking on veggies is a terrific strategy to help you control your appetite and maintain a healthy lifestyle.

Vegetables have so many wonderful qualities. It is surprising that they are so scarce in the average American diet. Walking around the exterior of your grocery store first is one of the greatest strategies to assist yourself to avoid high fat, high sugar, and high salt processed items.
Instead of rushing to the end and cheating by choosing pastas and other processed meals that are poor in actual nutritional vegetable content, go through the fresh produce area and make intentional decisions to provide your body with healthy fresh vegetable options.

Making the choice to fuel your body is the first step toward healthy eating, and few things are more nutritious than veggies.
We can often lose our taste for healthy foods because of unhealthy and poor eating habits early in life, or even self-imposed later in life, but it is easy to get back on track. Make time in your life for vegetables. They may take a little bit longer to prepare, but the

benefits are worth it.

CHAPTER 7: THE HEALTH BENEFITS OF FRUIT

People who follow the traditional American diet do not consume enough fruit, which is terrible but a common fact. What fruit they do consume is frequently canned or sugar-laden. The additional sugar and fruit detracts from any health benefits that consuming fruit in its natural condition might bring the body.

Eating too much fruit might lead to difficulties, especially if you have diabetes. Fruit is strong in natural sugars, and when juiced, you receive a lot of sugar without much fiber, which can overload the body.

The fruit's fiber content is one of its healthiest qualities, since it aids the body in lowering heart disease and avoiding constipation. Furthermore, fiber-rich foods such as fruits and vegetables are highly useful for weight control since they help you feel full of fewer calories. Not only that, but the fruit is abundant in numerous vitamins and minerals, particularly vitamin C-rich citrus fruits.

Vitamin C is a healing powerhouse, and if you're looking for anything to help you maintain your teeth and gums healthy, vitamin C-rich foods will undoubtedly do the work.

Another thing that fruit may do for the body is prevent strokes and kidney stones. Fruits are extremely beneficial to the body, preventing and treating diseases such as skin ailments and heart problems. Fruit may be one of the healthiest methods to improve your energy and eliminate sugar cravings that you may have when striving to eliminate bad items from your diet.

If you are ready to use the great power of fruit, you may have a nutritious snack that fulfills your sweet desire as long as you don't overdo it with your fruits, such as tossing a bunch of them in the blender and ultimately ingesting a ludicrous quantity of sugar.

If you're curious about the health advantages of eating, both fruits and vegetables have a natural propensity to make your skin glow and seem significantly more moisturized and nourished. Fruits and vegetables are abundant in antioxidants, vitamins, and minerals, which hydrate your body and keep your skin and look healthy.
It can help your hair grow softer and healthier, as well as keep your skin looking young. Fruit can even help you halt acne in its tracks by removing waste items from your body and moisturizing your skin. Because of its high water content, fruit is wonderful for helping the body keep hydrated, and you will rapidly notice the advantages and that aspect.

Not only that, but fruit is very good for digestion. Because of the high fiber content, it aids in the binding of waste and aids the body in eliminating substances that may otherwise create problems.
As a result, fruits and vegetables can also help with weight loss. Instead of allowing waste to be broken down and stored as fat, the body removes it before it can.

Fruit is another excellent strategy to fight and prevent disease, including cancer. Some foods, such as apples, can help prevent asthma attacks. Others have the ability to drastically decrease cholesterol levels.

Grapes, particularly red skinned grapes, have been utilized in the treatment of cancer. They are also beneficial in the treatment of eye and renal diseases. Berries are very beneficial if you have an illness. They contain a lot of antioxidants.
Just make sure to consume fruits and vegetables that have not been sprayed with commercial pesticides, since these chemicals can absorb and complicate weight reduction and cause difficulties

in the body.

You may also consume dry fruits to replace unhealthy and sugary snacks and provide your body with a sweet snack that packs a nutritious punch. Just be aware of the sugar levels in dried fruits, because when they are commercially offered, extra sugars can turn what might be a nutritious treat into something that will eventually help you gain weight.

Fruit, on the other hand, can help you lose weight if you consume it in a healthy and consistent manner. As long as you don't overeat sugary foods, the fibers and water content of fruit will keep your body full and your cells and organs fed. The fibers and water content will help you remove difficulties that contribute to obesity, and you will notice a significant improvement in your energy levels overall.

You may channel this enthusiasm into fitness and a healthier lifestyle. This is especially useful if you are replacing sugary junk meals with healthier fruit options as you continue on your path to greater health and well-being.

CHAPTER 8: HEALTHY LIVING WITH THE BEST MEAT

Meat is widely regarded as one of the most important staple items in an email, but it may surprise you to learn that some meats are really healthier than others. Of course, we understand the distinction between red and white meats. Red meat is more frequently associated with health concerns and cardiovascular disorders, whereas white meat is regarded leaner and better overall.

Some individuals may be shocked to learn that there are other factors that contribute to the harmful nature of meat. Issues such as what they are given while the animals are still living, as well as antibiotics and hormones put into them to make them grow faster or produce more milk, in the case of cows.

These hormones eventually make their way into the meat we eat and can create issues in our own bodies. If we are not diligent about the dietary choices we make, they can eventually lead to bad health in the future, including but not limited to tumors and hormone changes that can be fairly debilitating.

However, if you are satisfied that your meat is coming from a healthy source that does not overfeed animals with steroids and antibiotics, you are already ahead of the game. If not, attempt to find local businesses where you can get meat that hasn't been polluted by unsafe industrial standards.

Having said that, even among the healthy meat selections, there are some that are healthier than others. Fish is one of the healthiest meats you can consume, especially if you're trying to reduce weight. Fish is low in fat and high in nutrients. You must, however, be cautious about the source of your seafood.

Some fish are grown in poor conditions, while others may come from locations poisoned by mercury. This is why pregnant women should avoid eating fish or shellfish.
However, if you can locate a good supply of fish, it may be quite helpful to your body. Fish contains omega-3 fatty acids, which aid with brain function and memory. Overall, Omega three fatty acids are highly sought after, and the body needs them to perform at their peak, particularly in intellectual affairs.

Another excellent alternative is chicken produced in a healthy environment. Chicken has a lot of protein. In fact, it has the most protein of any meat. They are normally grown in decent circumstances, or are given meals that do not produce problems in the human body in the same way as a lot of beef does.
However, if you consume grass-fed beef from a reputable provider, it might also be a terrific alternative. If you consume organic chicken, there is a lower chance that these animals were grown with hazardous carcinogens.

Conventionally raised hens are typically fed meals that accelerate their growth, which can result in major health issues for both the chickens and the humans who consume them. They are also given an abundance of antidepressants and pain relievers, as well as arsenic and caffeine.
It is risky to consume a lot of conventionally raised beef, but if you can locate a decent provider, you should absolutely do so.

Another fantastic meat is turkey, which is high in selenium. This is beneficial to the body, especially because it can aid in the elimination of free radicals and other dangerous compounds.
Again, you should strive to get your meat from reputable sources because it is common for commercially farmed chicken and turkey to be treated identically and fed hazardous chemicals that unnaturally boost their rate of growth and eventually

contaminate human bodies with those chemicals.

Eating meat in general may be highly helpful to the body, as long as it is not from unsafe and traditionally cultivated techniques. The toxins that these creatures are frequently exposed to are extremely harmful, both to the animals and to the humans that consume them. If you want to eat healthily and lose weight, you should avoid any substances that may wind up lingering in your body and hinder weight loss.

Even if you don't want to lose weight, eating healthily means avoiding anything that might be harmful to your body, such as hormones and chemicals that upset our delicate systems. Fortunately, there are numerous options for healthy proteins, whether you prefer chicken, beef, or lamb. There are options for getting nutritious, ethically farmed meat to satisfy whatever needs you may have.

CHAPITRE 9: THE RISKS OF PROCESSED FOODS

It should come as no surprise that processed meals are hazardous. What is surprising is that they are still permitted on the market, despite the destruction they cause in our bodies and brains. Eating unhealthy food is more than simply a personal preference for some people.

People in poverty are often compelled to turn to processed meals because they are a cheap and quick way to feed big families on a limited budget.
The difficulty is that these meals eventually induce medical problems that cost much more money than it would take to feed a big family healthy, sustainable choices. In the end, it appears that individuals with little resources are suffering in either case.

Even if you don't have a family to feed, processed meals are plain bad. Their high fat and sugar content contribute to their addictive nature.
They are frequently packaged dinners with pasta and an excessive quantity of sugar. Excess sugar is hazardous in general, but it is especially risky for persons who are predisposed to type II diabetes. If you drink a lot of sugar, you will eventually overwhelm your body, and you will not only grow obese, but you will also have health problems.

Sugar can hasten the progression of diabetes because it increases insulin resistance, which makes controlling blood sugar levels difficult, if not impossible.

If you consume things like these frequently, such as at every meal or at least every day, there will be a detrimental effect. Consuming too much fat and sugar on a regular basis may lead to not just the well-known diabetes and obesity, but also heart disease and even cancer. This is extremely harmful, and processed meals should be avoided at all costs.

Another risk of eating processed meals is that they are not only addictive but also exceedingly unnatural. The majority of the elements in those foods are not beneficial to the body. Rather, they make us feel full while depriving our systems of crucial nutrients needed for optimum functioning.

When we consume a diet that is bland and devoid of nutrients, we are eventually dumbing ourselves down. We're not thinking clearly, we're not moving well, and we're not performing to our full capacity. All of these things are quite harmful and can result in poor coordination and even depression.

On some level, we all understand that processed meals are not as nutritious as the things we should eat on a daily basis. Our bodies are aware of it, even if our minds are not. And we pay the price. We're worried about it.

Our bodies know when we eat unhealthy foods, whether we are hooked on them or not. And, whether consciously or unconsciously, we frequently punish ourselves. We are well aware that we are making a mistake. Even though we are now digesting it, we are irritated and unsatisfied.

Artificial colorings, which have been shown to be very carcinogenic, are also abundant in processed foods. When we consume foods with fixed coloring, we are practically ingesting dye. Would you like to consume hair dye? Not at all. However, these are the compounds found in your diet. They remain in your body and do not leave. On the inside, they color your organs. They are extremely harmful and can cause cancer.

It's also loaded with preservatives. Processed food lasts a long time on the shelf longer than what is considered healthy and typical. A standard bottle of milk would not last for months on end. It would curdle and become bad. The same goes for cheeses and other items with a lengthy shelf life that you may find in stores.

Companies must set shelf life because they can make more money if their food can stay on the shelf for a longer period of time. They will do whatever it takes, whether it is healthy or not for the human body, to make the most money possible.
Preservatives sometimes contain harmful and unnatural compounds, as well as excessive levels of salt. Neither of which is beneficial for the body. Because of the high salt content in these meals, processed foods might induce cardiac problems and hypertension. High blood pressure is widespread among those who live on processed foods, and obesity and heart attacks are among the leading causes of death in North America.

This has everything to do with the typical American diet. The unfortunate issue is that even if you are aware that these processed meals are harmful, the chemicals and high sugar and fat content make them incredibly addictive.
The body develops a need for them, which may be as hazardous as a drug addiction. Addiction to a diet that is neither nourishing nor healthy can have long-term effects on your health and development.

Another way that processed meals contribute to obesity is that we digest them much faster than those high in beneficial dietary fiber. If we digest these meals fast and they do not fill us up because we are not getting the fiber that gives us a full sensation, we are not even using the same amount of energy to digest nutritious foods.
As a result, we consume more and digest less, which causes a quick and rapid weight gain. When you eat a lot of processed foods, your body contains far more calories. When you consume wholesome, high-dietary fiber meals, you burn a lot more calories.
Unfortunately, this means that whether they want to or not, people who eat a diet high in processed foods will eventually gain

weight. And because they are not nutritional, they won't provide you the same level of energy. Because you consume a lot more of these harmful, sugar-filled meals without feeling satisfied or exhausted, they are likely to make you feel sluggish, sleepy, and much too full.
Our bodies do not adequately digest processed foods. They swiftly develop into fat. Furthermore, they are high in fat. They are frequently high in hidden fat and sugar. Many of these processed meals contain vegetable oil as a significant component, as well as high fructose corn syrup, which is a major contributor to weight gain.

If every processed item on the market included high fructose corn syrup, as the vast majority do, it is no surprise that North America is experiencing the largest obesity pandemic in history. Hydrogenated oils are extremely harmful since they do not degrade.
They remain in your body and are absorbed by fat cells. These oils make fat burning much more difficult. They are more difficult to eliminate, and this sort of persistent fat can swiftly progress to obesity. The components in processed foods lack the majority of the nutritious content that humans require to function at their best. Before we can completely thrive, we require the fiber, vitamins, and minerals found in real food.

If processed foods cannot be avoided totally, they should be consumed in moderation. They are hazardous. They can make us feel lethargic, angry, and unsatisfied in general.
When we abandon a healthy diet in favor of manufactured foods that are too sweet, too fatty, and too unhealthy, our dispositions might shift from positive to negative.

Our bodies are hungry. Providing the fuel for your body is the simplest and most helpful thing you can do for yourself. It can be difficult to adjust to new patterns, such as relying on processed meals, and it can be extremely stressful at times.
You'll have to spend a lot more time in the kitchen preparing

and thinking about your health and food. But, in the end, consuming manufactured meals can kill you and cut you off from yourself. You are ingesting pollutants while avoiding foods that can function as antioxidants, giving you a chance to get rid of the garbage that you are putting into your body.

Processed foods are synonymous with junk foods. They are no exception. They appear to be healthier junk meals. Furthermore, they're actually nibbles. The first and most effective action you can take to get healthy and feel healthy is to avoid processed meals at all costs. Don't be misled by packaging that promises certain items are healthy.

They are high in saturated fat, sugar, and salt, and low in everything that nourishes your body. Make every effort to break your dependency on processed meals. Eating healthy is simple and achievable if you put your mind to it.

Remember the approach of wandering around the grocery store to get fresh vegetables and meat rather than walking through the aisles full of harmful and enticing packaging that hides the risks of the processed food within.

CHAPTER 10: MEAL PLANNING BRINGS IT ALL TOGETHER

One of the most crucial parts of adopting a healthy lifestyle is meal planning. When we are unable to see the future of our eating, it is all too easy to give in to the attractions of unhealthy foods to which we have been hooked. Especially if we have a habit of consuming them instead of things that feed us.
Meal preparation is a time-consuming task. It might be scary, especially for someone who struggles with organization. Don't worry if you're having trouble arranging your meals. Whether you struggle with creativity in the kitchen or not, there are many fun and easy ways to get started with meal planning.

You may purchase a variety of meal planning packages. Many of them provide the option of buying boxes full of fresh items to cook with, as well as recipes. This may be really beneficial if you are unfamiliar with cooking, which is frequently the case.

Especially when poor eating habits and a hectic work schedule make it appear impossible to find the time to prepare large, nutritional meals. Research is the first step in meal planning. If you want to get healthy, you need to consider your alternatives.
The best way to begin is by researching recipes. Creating a binder full of nutritious meals to try may be both entertaining and instructive. It will open your eyes to various meal options that you might have dismissed as too difficult for you to cook, or it may teach you something you didn't know before.

Recipes may be quite enlightening. Especially if you're looking to make fresh discoveries. Cooking might be a difficult habit to develop, but once you do, you will be astonished at how much freedom you can discover in preparing a dinner for yourself that is both healthy and tasty!

Look through recipe books and periodicals for recipes that you wish to try. Beginning with what appears to be the most tasty and nourishing, and if you are a newbie in the kitchen, you may also want to consider what appears to be the most straightforward.

Next, keep your recipes arranged in a basic, easy-to-navigate format. Meal preparation will be more difficult if you are overwhelmed by a lack of structure.

When starting a new habit, you want to make sure that everything is as simple as possible. Too much change at once may be taxing on your system, so always strive to make tiny, simple adjustments until they become a new habit.

Make sure they are conveniently accessible so that you can begin cooking your dinner as soon as possible. If you use a binder, consider laminating the pages or using plastic sleeves so that they are not harmed by water or other food contamination if you use it in the kitchen.

When organizing your recipes, place them in the sequence of breakfast meals, lunch meals, dinner meals, and snacks. This will make it easier for you to find the right recipes once you start cooking. You could even organize your binder by weekday and have your meals planned out for each day and written out in the binder that way.

There are several ways to arrange your recipes. Do what naturally makes the most sense to you. Don't push yourself to be a part of an organization that doesn't suit you. Instead, make sure you're doing what's best for you in your own life.

Make it a habit to search out new recipes that stand out to you on a regular basis to keep your creative juices flowing and your kitchen intriguing. There are several recipes to explore, and the more you try, the more enjoyable embarking on a healthy eating journey may be!

Next, look at tools such as Excel in Microsoft Office to assist you with your food planning. Excel has a wealth of templates from which to choose to help you plan out your meals by day, time, and week. This may be a really useful resource!
If you don't want to use Excel, there are apps you can download on your phone, tablet, or other device to help you better manage your time and resources.

You may also go the traditional approach and purchase a notebook specifically intended for meal planning. This is a critical step in ensuring that your meals are organized and easily available.

When going on a journey of healthy eating, having a meal plan is tremendously beneficial. Developing excellent habits requires time and patience, and you will inevitably mess up sometime along the road.
But it doesn't mean you have to remain on the ground! Actually, it just means that you must get back up and try again, because giving up is much easier than sticking to your intentions.

Sticking to a theme may be really beneficial when it comes to meal planning. Many people, for example, have certain themes, such as taco Tuesday or another day designated for a specific style of cuisine. Feel free to mimic that style of menu planning if you believe it would help you remain on track. It is done for a reason: it works and aids in keeping things simple and streamlined.
It may be really inconvenient to be stuck doing a lot of planning and preparation every week or month, so if you want to keep things simple, this can be a smart way to go. You may have a bimonthly dinner theme, such as taco Tuesday one night and rice and veggies Tuesday the next, and rotate between them. There is no such thing as a bad approach to arranging your meals. What

you must ensure is that you observe and follow through.
Without follow-through, everything else becomes superfluous and difficult. Meal planning is something that may genuinely help you succeed at meal planning. If you tell someone you love and care about that you're trying to organize your meals, ask them if they'd be willing to assist you in keeping to your pattern.

They can assist you by inquiring about how things are going and whether or not you are on track. They may also choose to encourage and support you in your attempts.

They may be incredibly gratifying for both of you, whatever they choose to assist you with. If they are positive and supportive individuals, it might be reassuring to know that you have people on your side who genuinely want you to succeed. Just make sure you're weeding out toxic people who pull you down by drawing attention to themselves or making you believe it would be tough to achieve your objectives.

Sure, constructive comments may be quite beneficial, but if you are not actively seeking them, they can be poisonous at times. Make sure you know the difference between a poisonous individual masquerading as a support person and a supportive person who genuinely wants you to succeed.

Personal accountability is another method of accepting accountability. Personal accountability can be helped by journaling and self-affirmation. Talking to yourself about your objectives, what you do internally or out loud, may help you stay focused and ask yourself if you are doing the things you want to do.

If you discover that you are not, instead of berating yourself, analyze your difficulties and move on as you uncover them. The only way you will ever fail is if you never try. Everything will eventually fall into place if you try since you are putting an effort into making great changes in your life.

Journaling is beneficial for a variety of reasons. They can assist you in writing down what you ate, when you ate it, and how much you ate. This will give you a decent notion of what you may realistically anticipate from yourself. Things you are dissatisfied with should be addressed and noted. But, rather than becoming irritated with yourself for not becoming a trickle right away, realize that it is a process and that you must go gently.

Instead of imposing a complete shift in routine and planning out every meal for the next month if you have never done it before, begin cautiously by easing into one or two meals each week and gradually adding in the rest as you feel comfortable with the process.

Make it something that will not startle you. The greatest long-lasting change is gradual transformation. And blogging about your experiences can assist you in uncovering your innermost feelings about the process as well as things that you may not have realized were holding you back.

You will begin to notice patterns in your conduct and may be able to forecast when and why you might be tempted to stray. It will be easier to avoid these trigger points in the future if you can recognize them.

Meal preparation can be a lot of fun and thrilling. Even if you're not the sort that appreciates that kind of organization, it can be incredibly fulfilling to consider exactly what you're going to put in your body and take the required measures to do so. Everyone deserves the opportunity to become the healthiest and most healthy version of themselves, and with meal planning and a good dose of self-esteem, you will be well on your way to a healthy eating habit.

PART TWO : HEALTHY VEGETARIAN

CHAPTER 1: HOW TO BECOME A VEGETARIAN.

It may seem impractical to imagine the initiatives a person must take to learn to transition to a vegetarian diet. However, eliminating meat from your diet is not that easy. The answer to this simple problem is... not really.

People realize that going vegan takes a lot more effort than just turning down a steak or burger. A person would find that trying to go vegan takes a lot of testing and also some serious effort to get fit. and not be without something it essentially needs to function as designed. The most important thing to try when transitioning to a vegan diet is to take it slow. for years, in which case a relaxed attitude won't matter much. You need to make some serious and planned efforts to become a vegan.

Start by gradually eliminating meat from your regular diet. You can reduce meat for a few days and then switch to fish or chicken. This process can help you wean yourself off meat permanently as your body adjusts to it slowly and gradually. to change diet. If a person wants to know how to follow a lacto vegetarian diet, then they must also do a little research into the nutrients contained in various vegetables so that a person can be sure that their body is getting the essential material it needs to be well built and efficient. It should be noted that vitamins such as B and C and minerals such as iron and zinc are essential to human life.

Calcium and protein are also important components of a balanced diet, so you want to know the nutritional value of the foods you eat. It must be ensured that the body is getting all the essential nutrients and vitamins it needs. required to function efficiently.

As people eliminate meat from their diets, they need to make sure they're getting enough protein in their bodies. Therefore, when people learn how to go vegan, they will want to have backup supplies. of protein so your body can function the way it was designed.

Eating a Healthy Vegetarian

Although vegan diets are known to be very healthy and filling, they generally attract little extra attention when a person is vegetarian. When a person avoids red meat and animal protein from their diet, they are avoiding an important source of protein that their body needs. It means that eating healthy as a vegan involves adding foods to the diet that provide the nutrients commonly found in meat products. By exploring a diet comprised of

fruits, vegetables, and whole grains, people can easily get the vitamins and nutrients they need from vegetarian sources to keep their vegetarian lifestyle healthy and appropriate.

By consuming foods like legumes, soy products, nuts and eggs, one can get the essential protein content one needs for the diet. Other nutrients such as the minerals iron, calcium and vitamins D and B12 are just as important for vegans. It is a fact that eliminating meat from your diet and consuming a diet rich in vegetables, fruits and grains is healthy. and minerals from your diet. Many may take vitamin supplements regularly, but since many of these supplements contain animal derivatives, many devout vegetarians are reluctant to take them.

It is important to strive for a diet rich in vitamins B and C, iron and niacin, as these are also an essential part of a healthy lacto-vegetarian lifestyle. If you eat vegan, you don't have to sacrifice your health. Eating a healthy vegetarian diet is no easy task. One should only take free time to study and find foods that contain the most important nutrients for the body. extensively consult various books and magazines or even surf the Internet.

People can make all sorts of changes to their diet that can replace meat when they stop eating. For example, you can opt for soy milk as an alternative to cow's milk, which in turn provides the body with the calcium it needs. Including nuts and grains in a vegetarian diet makes it a healthy diet. Nuts and grains are also packed with proteins that help build healthy bones. Various studies have shown that vegetarians generally have a healthy diet that leads to a healthy and fit body.

They are also more likely to stay healthy and energetic. What people need to keep in mind for a healthy vegan diet is that they need to pay special attention to the nutritional content of the food and eat a balanced diet.

CHAPTER 2: VEGETARIAN DIET FOR WEIGHT LOSS

Many people choose to become vegetarian because they need to diet to lose weight, but hate the idea of starving themselves.

Eliminate all red meat, which can be high in fat that is stored in your body cells and actually causes you to gain weight. A vegetarian eats lots of fruits and vegetables as well as fish and shellfish, which are healthy for you and can be a great way to lose weight. Dieting is difficult because you want to achieve your weight loss goal, so you really want to consider making a change of the vegetarian lifestyle.

Vegetables are naturally low in calories and good for you, so you don't have to worry about gaining weight. Although fruit is good for you, it contains a lot of water and can make you weigh more as the body tends to retain water, but know that you're still eating healthy. A good, balanced vegetarian diet for maximum weight loss includes a variety of foods and spices that taste good and help you feel full. You see, food makes you fat because of how we prepare it and what we add to it. You can have a bowl full of healthy mushrooms, but if you cook them in butter and add some cream to make a soup, you've piled on the calories. and negated the naturally healthy effects.

If you are following a vegetarian diet for weight loss, avoid deep frying your food as much as possible. If you want to sauté some of your veggies, do so in extra virgin olive oil (or EVOO, as Rachel Ray says), which is lower in calories and provides some of the good fats your body needs. You should also steer clear of high-fat cheeses and opt for lower-fat varieties and try substitutes like using plain yogurt. for the sour cream. A vegetarian diet is an excellent means of weight loss as well as a healthy diet. Once you've reached your weight loss goals, we're happy to bet you'll stick to your vegetarian diet.

Giving up meat is not as difficult as many think. You'll find that you have more energy, a faster metabolism (which burns fat), and lower grocery bills, especially if you grow most of your veggies. Go vegan for maximum weight loss and watch the pounds melt away without feeling hungry all the time.

CHAPTER 3: BEING A VEGETARIAN

Being a vegetarian is a great way to stay healthy. Not only does it help kickstart your metabolism, but it ultimately leads to a much healthier lifestyle. We often see people around us who need to adopt proper nutrition because of a disease they may have contracted as a result of improper diet. Since carnivores are more prone to cholesterol build-up and diabetes, being a vegetarian could help them stay in proper control of their health.

If we look at vegetarians in general, one might think that these people eat a lot of green salad, but this view is somewhat wrong, as the classification from a broader perspective is very different from what is considered. Here are some classifications: • Lacto-Ovo-Vegetarian - People who prefer to eat both dairy products and eggs. This is the diet most commonly preferred by vegetarians.

• Lacto-Vegetarian - Under this category, people consume dairy products but not eggs.

• Vegan: People who do not consume dairy, eggs, or animal products. • Frugivore: Categorized as vegan, this is a classification where consumption of processed foods is minimized to optimal levels. It consists mainly of raw fruits, grains and nuts. Since frugivores believe in only eating food that can be harvested without killing the plant. • Macrobiotic: This type of diet is followed for spiritual and philosophical reasons.

It is viewed in terms of the negative and positive energies that food contains. Yin is the positive attribute while yang is the negative attribute. This style of eating aims to maintain adequate nutrition. ten levels it is reduced. The entire level includes vegetarians, but ultimately eliminates animal products and, in extreme cases, even fruits and vegetables, resulting in a diet consisting entirely of brown rice.

Everyone has their own reasons why they chose to go vegetarian, for a much healthier alternative. The reason could be anything, but it has also been medically proven that vegetarians are much healthier. Vegetarians are less prone to cholesterol build-up, diabetes, and even eliminate the risk of some cancers.

Organic Foods are grown with minimal use of pesticides, eliminating the risk of consuming harmful chemicals that scientists have shown seriously damage the proper functioning of the body and nervous system. If that somehow convinced you to become a vegetarian, then take a step towards a much healthier life.

In the beginning it could be very exhausting and difficult, but in the long run it would bring about drastic changes that would lead to much safer and better health.

CHAPTER 4: VEGETARIAN SPORTS NUTRITION

Suppose you exercise a lot but eat vegan and are concerned about proper nutrition.

Don't worry. You can get all the nutrients you need while still being a vegetarian. lifestyle and physical activity. You don't have to cut back on your diet just because you don't want to eat meat.

In fact, you may find that a vegetarian diet is very conducive to participating in exercise as the nutrients found in vegetables, fruits and grains will actually give you more energy.

The first thing you should do is remember to eat before you train so your body can start processing food and provide you with the nutrients you need to sustain a heavy workout and have enough energy. to participate in the sports you love. This means that vegetarians should eat plenty of carbohydrates before exercise and then let the nutrients found in these high-carb foods work for you. You also need to eat a good vegetarian meal after exercise so you can replenish the nutrients that are naturally lost through sweat during exercise. However, you should avoid carbohydrates in this meal as much as possible, as carbohydrates are easily converted to fat and will negate any benefit you have just given yourself.

If you exercise a lot and are lacto-vegetarian, we recommend consuming lots of nuts and grains, which are full of carbohydrates, as well as lots of fruit, which can give your body something it needs. Water that is eventually sweated out during sports training.

Athletes who follow a vegetarian diet often worry about their diet as exercise is very important to staying fit. All you really need to remember is that the body needs certain vitamins and minerals to function properly. That's where research comes in. Ask some of your vegetarian friends what they do before exercise so their diet doesn't suffer.

Search online for tips on what to do to get the most out of your vegetarian diet before you exercise. Read books and consult your doctor. if you have diet concerns as a vegetarian who exercises frequently. As the old saying goes, you can never have enough information, so find out what's in it for you and then pay attention. It will be worth it in the end!

CHAPTER 5: VEGETARIAN COOKING FOR ALL

Vegetarian cooking is one of the easiest things to learn. Even those who are afraid of boiling water or cooking food will find vegetarian food very interesting and easy to prepare. Vegetarian cuisine is something for everyone. Not only does it have high nutritional value, but vegetarian cooking is easy for everyone.

For people who are vegan and enjoy preparing gourmet meals, there are tremendous opportunities to explore and find. There are a large number of delicious vegan recipes that a person can prepare in different places and in different situations; You just have to search for prospects to do this.

We'll start first with, which defines an Epicurean meal.

Now the question arises whether this is feasible. Actually, a gourmet meal is a special meal without meat or spaghetti and involves transforming interesting and rare items into masterpieces that are not only delicious but also remarkable looking. Of course, gourmet food can be explained in many different ways by many people, but cooking a gourmet vegan meal takes enough talent. It takes great taste and skill to turn simple ingredients into artistic creations. So, what do you need to know to prepare a gourmet vegetarian meal?

If you've been a lacto-vegetarian for a while, you might want to share ideas about what people love to eat and how to innovate to make it unusual and delicious as well as appetizing. When people are new to vegetarian cooking, it's best to consider the types of gourmet meals they've had before. It is very true that almost every one of us has eaten vegetarian at some point. Avoid the meat portion on the plate while leaving the essence intact. With a little brains and ingenuity this is possible, we know almost anyone can do it!

An individual can find vast and varied cookbooks dedicated solely to gourmet vegetarian cooking in their local bookstore, on various websites, and online. Browse through cooking methods that include components that will intrigue everyone, then try the recipe. Many won't be able to cook a gourmet vegetarian feast if they start anywhere. But if you strictly follow the instructions, you can avoid a gastronomic failure. never as a vegan cook.

Many people believe that the vegetarian lifestyle is one of confusion and curiosity. If it's easy to demonstrate that serving up a vegetarian feast is epicurean, flashy, and delicious, you might just be swayed to their side of the border. But don't try too hard. Being lacto vegetarian is not for everyone. The best thing people can do is cook from the heart and stay true to their commitment to a vegetarian lifestyle, which means cooking gourmet dishes that taste like lamb, even though they have no meat at all.

CHAPTER 6: LOW-CARB VEGETARIANS

The human body needs a variety of nutrients to stay fit. Being a vegetarian is good, but you need to be adept at balancing vitamins and nutrients. The only thing you need to be aware of is the carbohydrate balance. Carbs are a great source of energy and that's the only reason to eat carbs in the right proportions.

Excess carbohydrates in a vegetarian diet stimulate the production of fat in the human body. Carbohydrates break down sugars, which in turn are converted to fat, and this creates a problem when the amount converted is too high. Some foods like rice, potatoes, and grains are high in carbohydrates. So if you plan to reduce your carbohydrate intake, you should minimize your intake of these foods. It is also not recommended to completely eliminate these foods from your diet as they are a good source of carbohydrates. Efforts should be made to reduce consumption of these foods.

Carbohydrates are also found in flour, which includes whole wheat flour. You should avoid or minimize the consumption of bread if you are serious about adequate carbohydrate intake. Make sure your carbohydrate source is appropriate to monitor adequate intake. of carbohydrates. Stay away from white bread and eat whole grain bread to balance the body's carbohydrate needs. Being a vegetarian is good, but you have to give up a lot.

Your diet should include plenty of fresh, green vegetables. The selection of oils for the preparation of the food must also be considered. When using olive oil, you need to use the right amount to achieve the required carbohydrate content. Consider oil steaming and grilling to ensure low carb intake. It has the natural vitamins found in green and leafy vegetables.

Don't eat carbohydrates that make you gain weight. Different people have different reasons for changing their lifestyle to be vegetarian. The simplest reason is to lose extra weight. Some people are also very concerned about killing multiple animals. A balanced diet is the most important criterion for a vegetarian lifestyle.

Too much carbohydrate can be converted to sugar, which can eventually lead to extra weight gain. Before following a low-carb vegetarian diet, you need to be very careful to find the exact amount of carbohydrates in your diet. .If the amount of carbohydrates is too low, it can affect your body and, more importantly, your health. The most important part of a healthy diet is nutrition.

Low Calorie Vegetarian Recipes

Perhaps a person would have preferred a vegetarian lifestyle because they want to lose weight and need a low calorie vegan approach to achieve their weight loss goal. switch to meatless food; one would eat fewer calories. The undisclosed aspect of preparing healthy vegan recipes is removing the extra flab that makes meals filling. When a person prepares low-fat vegan recipes, the first thing they want to do is avoid using oil.

However, an individual can use a superior quality extra virgin olive oil for tastings and salads. EVOO is lower in calories and provides some of the "useful fats" our bodies need. Avoid fried foods while preparing vegetarian recipes that are lower in calories. Even when using the added extra virgin olive oil for frying, fried foods are still characteristically higher in calories, so fried foods should be avoided whenever possible. Alternatively, steam vegetables and do without cooking.

Boiling uses up important nutrients. Grill the vegetables to change them up. You can also apply a light or no-calorie cooking spray to moisten them a little, or even drizzle them with some watery lemon juice. If the diet allows you to eat shellfish. Cook the fish while you fry it. Grilling fish is recommended as grilling is a great way to add flavor and elegance to your meals.

Spices are the key ingredients that can make all the difference, delivering a low-fat vegetarian recipe that's both enjoyable and delicious. You can find many recipes for low-calorie vegetarian meals online. A person can also buy vegan cookbooks with low-fat recipes in them. A more convenient and effortless way to prepare low-calorie vegetarian recipes is to simply change up the usual recipes by using healthy substitutes like diet cheese or substituting sour cream for plain yogurt. If a person is creative, they will. Be surprised to discover that you can discover many healthy vegetarian recipes and use these recipes in the diet that balances your weight loss goals.

All a person needs is a little learning where to make substitutions that will turn high calorie foods into light foods with a little variation and a lot of thought. Incorporate low calorie vegan recipes into your daily eating plan and know that you can eat tasty foods while maintaining your meatless standard of living.

CHAPTER 7: VEGAN VEGETARIANS

The difference between vegetarians and non-vegetarians is well known as the eating habits are different and obvious. There is another branch of the food group that is commonly known as vegan, and the difference between vegetarian and vegan is often misunderstood. There is no surprising difference between vegan and vegetarian eating habits, but still people get confused when categorizing these food groups. As a layman you will not be able to understand the difference between vegan and vegetarian.

People think of them as the same food groups because the similarities are obvious and clear. People believe what they see, and you often see a vegetarian eating fresh green salads and little broccoli for all three meals. The fact is that different vegans and vegetarians consume foods very differently and their forms are not always similar. Understanding the eating habits of this faction will clear things up. Here are some examples.

People who consume dairy products, eggs, fruits and vegetables are classified as ovo lacto vegetarians. It is one of the most common types of lacto-vegetarian diets. There are instances where these groups eat fish and they also consume poultry products. Lacto-Vegetarian: Your diet includes vegetables, healthy nuts, fruits, grains, and dairy products. The only difference is the consumption of eggs, which this group avoids.

Vegan: The difference between vegans and vegetarians can be understood by their eating habits. Vegans do not include dairy, eggs or any kind of animal products in their regular diet. These vegans do not only do without sport or animal products.

Macrobiotics: There are many reasons to follow a group diet. The diet followed for philosophical and spiritual reasons is called the macrobiotic diet.

Health factors are also considered before selecting this diet. In this diet, foods are divided into negative and positive foods. The positive group is ying and the negative group is yang. There are stages of progression in this type of diet. The renunciation of animal products is encouraged at all levels.

The highest level even eliminates fruits and vegetables and is limited to brown rice. A normal person will definitely get confused between lacto-vegetarian and vegetarian diets. But for vegans and vegetarians it is quite easy to follow their lifestyle. As you begin to follow a diet, learn the pros and cons.

You should support all diet groups and eating habits to the extent that they are healthy and keep you strong.

CONCLUSION

Healthy eating might be tough to start, especially if you were not able to build healthy eating habits from an early age. It is, nevertheless, not difficult to become a more health-conscious and proactive individual.

Fortunately, every day that we wake up alive and breathing is a new opportunity to better ourselves and go ahead in our lives.
Being the greatest version of ourselves may seem daunting at first, but once you realize that every decision you make has an influence on your life, whether positive or negative, it becomes much simpler to see the path of our actions before they come back to haunt us. Poor eating habits are unquestionably bad decisions that will come back to haunt us.
We will acquire health problems later in life if we are not careful since we were not attentive of what we put into our bodies when we were younger. The only way to get a healthy and happy body and mind is via proper nutrition and exercise.

We feel bored and restless when we are cooped up in our houses all day, consuming only sugar and fat-laden manufactured meals and sitting around watching TV without moving. The typical American diet is hazardous and is costing people their lives. Don't allow yourself to become one of them.
Instead, make the necessary decisions to actually enhance yourself and become the best version of yourself possible. Make decisions that will make your family proud and ensure your presence in their lives for many years to come.

When we do not take care of ourselves, we are being really selfish. People around us, whether we realize it or not, care greatly about the people we are and the value we offer to their lives. Everyone deserves the opportunity to shape their own destiny and make constructive decisions that will benefit them for years to come.
Healthy eating is only one of many strategies to start bettering yourself and preparing your mind and body for the future. If you want to stay independent and active for as long as possible without spending thousands of dollars on medical bills and other costs, you should start eating healthy sooner rather than later.

Otherwise, it will become a burden on your life, both financially and physically. You are now better equipped to take the first step toward a healthy lifestyle after reading this book and using the ideas contained inside it.
Planning your meals and becoming more aware of why making healthy food choices is vital can enhance your quality of life now and in the future. All you have to do is stick with it, and you will immediately notice the benefits of good eating! All you have to do is give it a go. You've got this!

BOOKS BY THIS AUTHOR

Colouring Art Collection Anti-Stress For Children: Colouring Art Collection Anti-Stress Paperback

Experience a fun and whimsical fantasy adventure with this delightful children coloring book!
Would you want to unwind and appreciate line art designs? Looking for a fresh, original coloring book to inspire your imagination and give you the chance to practice mindfulness? Then you should read this book!
This book has something for everyone thanks to the fantastical mushrooms and toadstools, vibrant and exciting scenes, and loads of animals as well.
Coloring book information

70 hand-drawn illustrations specifically created to inspire your creative aspirations
Printed on separate sheets to avoid bleed-through and make it simple for you to remove and frame your favorites!
suitable for watercolors, colored pencils, fine-liners, gel pens, markers, and gel pens
Every skill level is catered for with a variety of easy and complicated drawings, and there are endless hours of coloring fun and mental relaxation.
So this book is for you if you're seeking for a silly and enjoyable fantasy journey to help you get lost in the world of coloring!

Amazing Nutritional And Veggie Power

This book describes in detail the importance of fruits and vegetables and how they contribute to your wellness.
The most typically recognized fat soluble vitamins are vitamin A, vitamin D, vitamin E and vitamin K.

Being fat soluble, it is saved inside the body and might assist to defend frame cells from the outcomes of loose radicals, which might be unfavorable to different body cells.

If your food regimen is deficient in the sort of nutrients, even for a short time, you can go through signs and symptoms of vitamin deficiency as a result, there may be no back up supply stored for your body.

While fruits are generally filled with vitamins, minerals generally tend to come more from our vegetables — although make no mistake, each fruit and vegetable are packed with both.

As well as being rich in vitamins and minerals, fruits and vegetables are also a wealthy source of the two other essential vitamins.
Do you want to have an understanding of the first-rate methods to get those fruits and veggies on your eating regimen, and the satisfactory methods to keep away from any troubles that can come from them.?
If you say yes, then this book is for you.

www.ingramcontent.com/pod-product-compliance
Lightning Source LLC
LaVergne TN
LVHW050344160826
845677LV00014B/3775